Table of Contents

About the author

My Health Record

Diseases & Symptoms	Recovered or not	Date
Cervical Carcinoma in Situ(CIS)	✓	Jun 2008
Hepatitis B (HBsAg-positive)	✓	Aug 1992
Thalassemia	✗	✗
Fibroadenoma of Breast	✓	Oct 1996
Poor Blood Circulation	✓	Aug 2005
Dry Eye	✓	Jan 2015
Dry Skin	✓	Nov 2011
Dyshidrotic Eczema	✓	Aug 2014
Rheumatoid Arthritis	✓	Aug 2002
Hot Flushes	✓	May 2018
Nocturnal Polyuria	✓	Apr 2018
Periodontal disease	✓	May 2018

Remarks :~

1. Thalassemia is a kind of inherited blood disorder that cannot be cured.

2. Through eyeball exercise, my Dry eye has been cured three years ago.

3. Doing sports and exercises makes my dry skin improve a great deal.

4. Practicing qigong for three months, I found my hot flushes begins to disappear.

5. Qigong also cured my nocturnal polyuria and I don't need to wake and pass urine at night now.

FORDWORD

Since I was a little girl, I have often experienced waking up with ankle or finger joints swelling and aching. My father, who was a doctor, told me that I should do exercises regularly for my entire life. It is because while sleeping, poor blood circulation sometimes will prevent blood from flowing to my distal extremities.

Until I was in my 30s, I realized that I had inherited my mother's Thalassemia. That is an inherited blood disorder that reduces the production of functional hemoglobin. I followed my father's suggestion, and since then doing exercises have become an integral part of my life.

Although exercising regularly did benefit most of my life, I must confront with the challenges of many different symptoms and diseases due to the inherited Thalassemia.

That is why I have been following closely to the latest health messages, especially after I got Cervical Carcinoma in 2004. Over these years, I found that creating good habits now really can get good health later.

Since I have been persevering to all those good habits, I found myself getting healthier day by day. Interpreting about my own experiences and feelings, I am convinced that I should be one of the most appropriate people to share all these abundance with you.

1) Stretch in bed

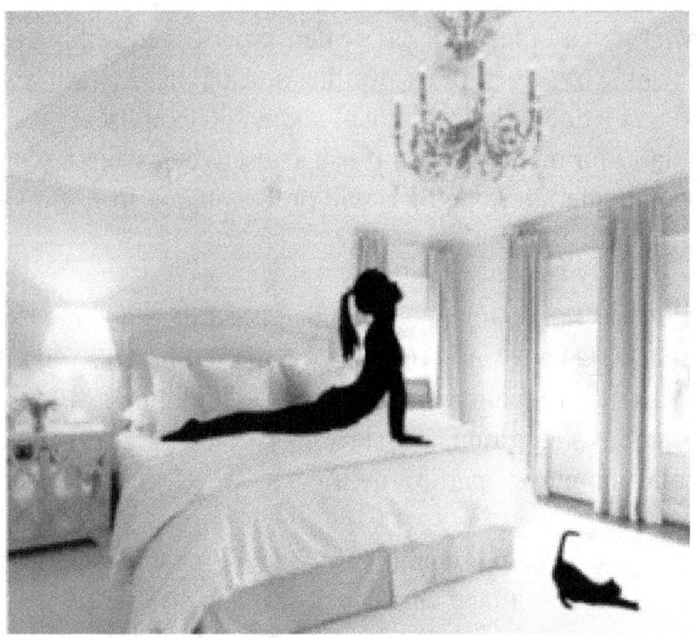

I will do some stretching to relax and protect my spine every morning. It can correct and strengthen my spine by doing these stretching exercises in bed before getting up.

Stretching exercise ~ Move like a caterpillar

- ➢ 1. Lie on your back.
- ➢ 2. Hands up.
- ➢ 3. Feet and toes down.

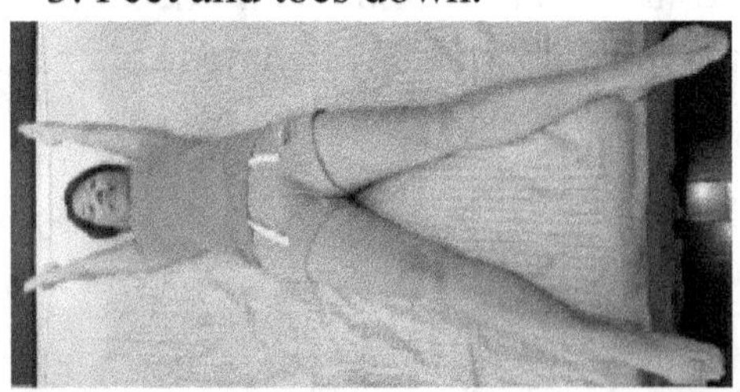

> ➢ 4. Stretching your right hand and right leg while squeezing your left pelvis and left shoulder towards your waist.
> ➢ 5. Stretching your left hand and left leg while squeezing your right pelvis and right shoulder towards your waist.

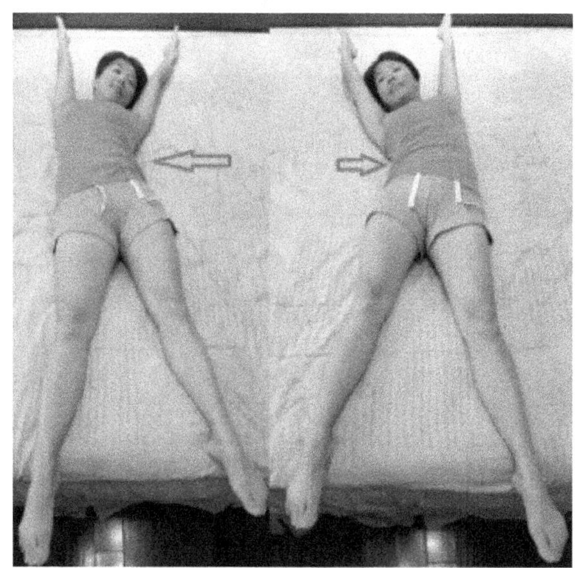

> ➢ 6. Repeat 4 ~ 5 and moving just like a caterpillar for 1 to 2 minutes.

Remarks:
This exercise can correct your spine, stretch your back, and improve cardiopulmonary function.

Stretching exercise ~ Legs swinging

> ➢ 1. Lie on your back with your head hanging over the bed edges.
> ➢ 2. With your arms hanging over your head and clench your hands.

➢   3. Knees bent, feet with shoulder width apart.

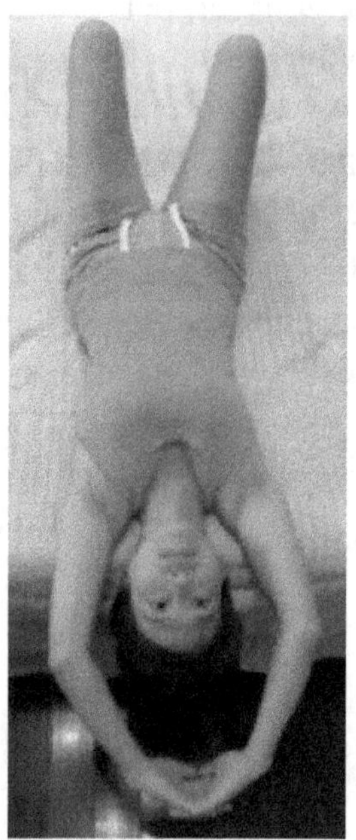

(Caution: If the above position causes dizziness, then your head should be on the bed instead of hanging over the bed edge.)

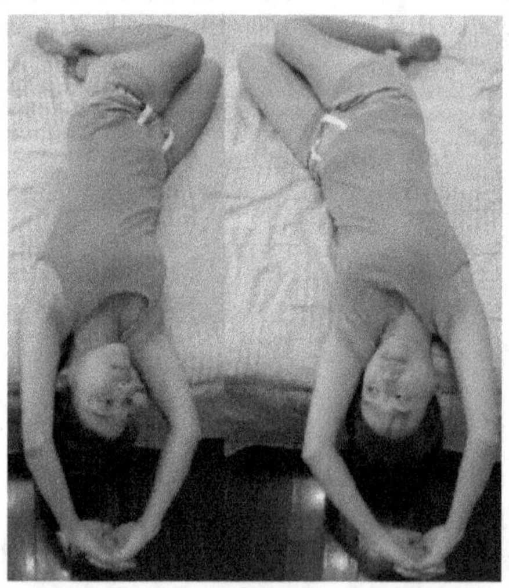

>   4. Knees together, and then turn your knees, your legs and your pelvis to the right side, with your right knee touching on the bed.
>   5. Turn back to the left side, with your left knee touching on the bed.
>   6. Repeat 4 ~ 5 for 50 ~ 100 times.

Remarks:
This exercise can correct your spine, reduce intracranial pressure, and improve cardiopulmonary function.

2) Exercise your eyes

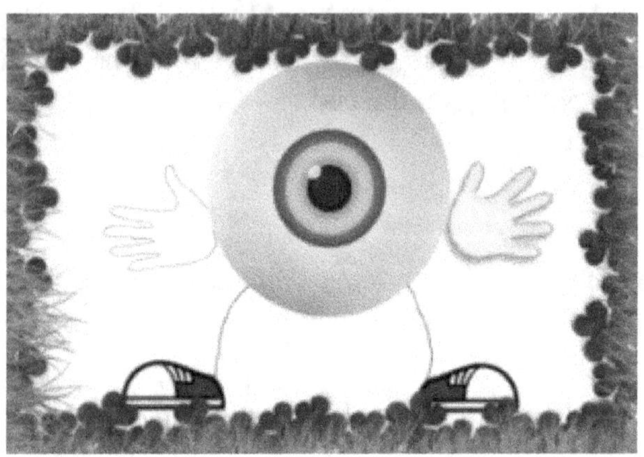

From around age 45, I started to get the following eye problems:

> Presbyopia ~ a kind of age-related loss of near focusing ability
> Dry eye ~ unable to secretes tears and fluid normally
> Eye discharge ~ a yellowish, sticky substance in eyes
> Sore eyes after reading ~ feel tired, heavy and hard to keep open.

Eyes exercises:

1. To relieve Dry eye:
   ~ Gently hold your eyelids open with your index finger and your thumb.

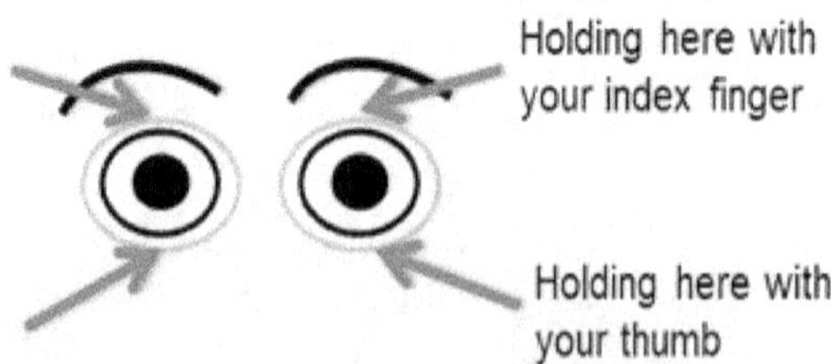

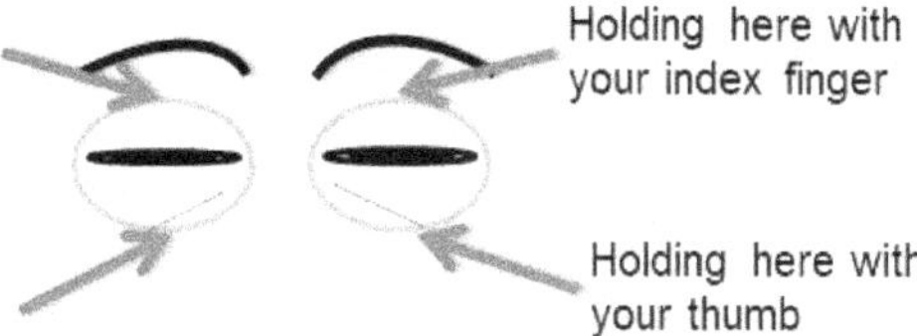

~ Slowly blink your eyes for 10 times, with eyelids
 opening.

~ Pull up the two ends of your eyes with your index
 fingers.

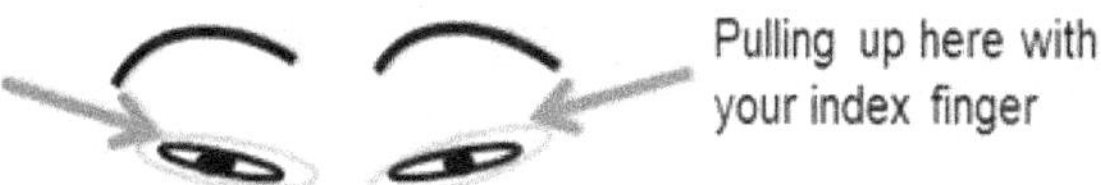

~ Slowly blink your eyes for 10 times, with eyes
 pulling up.

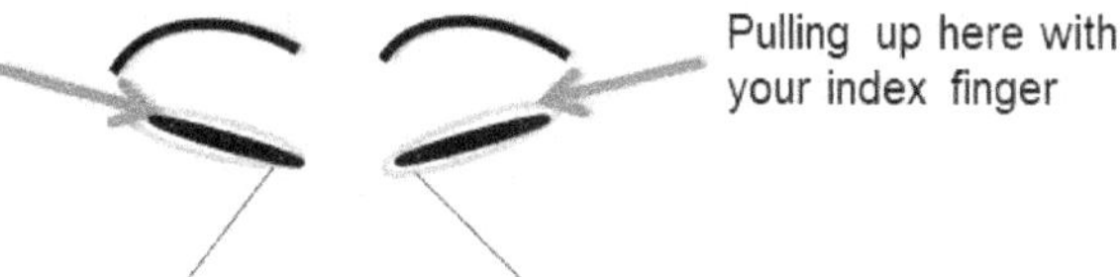

2. To relieve eye discharge:
 ~ Put your thumb about 30cm ahead of your nose and
   focus your eyes on your thumb.
 ~ Move your thumb forwards your nose and keep on
   focusing to form a cross-eye.
 ~ Slowly move your thumb back and forth for 10
   times.

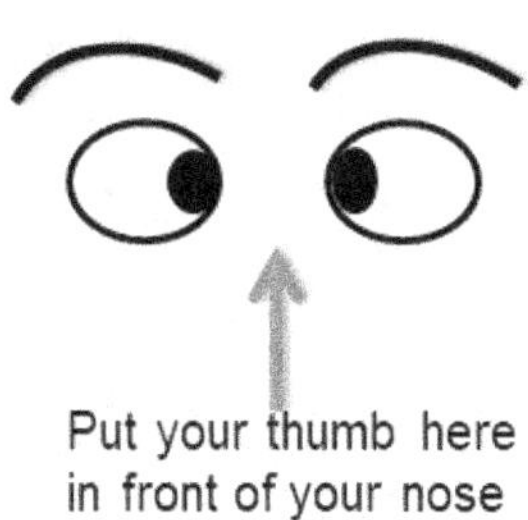

~ Put your thumb about 30cm ahead of your nose
  and focus your eyes on your thumb.
~ Swaying your thumb from left to right for 30 times,
  with your eyes following.

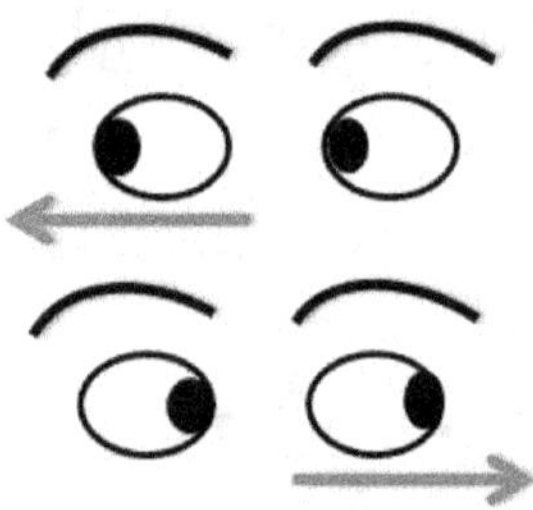

~ Swaying your thumb up and down for 30 times.

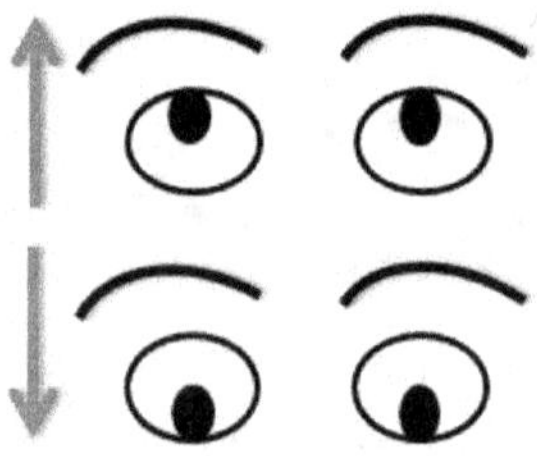

~ From lower left to upper right for 30 times.
~ From upper right to lower left for 30 times.

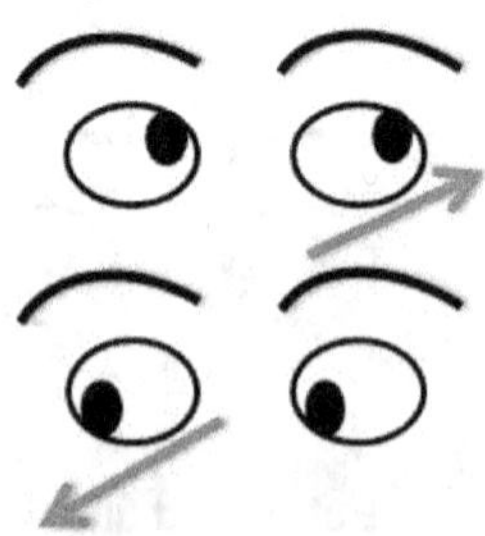

3. To relieve sore eyes:
  ~ Alternately winking your eyes:

<table>
<tr><td>

Counting 1 while winking your right eye
Count 3
Count 5
.
.

</td><td>

Counting 2 while winking your left eye
Count 4
Count 6
.
.

</td></tr>
<tr><td>

Counting 1,2 while winking your right eye twice
Count 3,2
Count 5,2
.
.

</td><td>

Count 2,2 while winking your left eye twice
Count 4,2
Count 6,2
.
.

</td></tr>
<tr><td>

Count 1,2,3 while winking your right eye 3 times
Count 3,2,3
Count 5,2,3
.
.

</td><td>

Count 2,2,3 while winking your left eye 3 times
Count 4,2,3
Count 6,2,3
.
.

</td></tr>
<tr><td>

Count 1,2,3,4 while winking your right eye four times
Count 3,2,3,4
Count 5,2,3,4
.
.

</td><td>

Counting 2,2,3,4 while winking your left eye four times
Count 4,2,3,4
Count 6,2,3,4
.
.

</td></tr>
</table>

  ~ by counting 1 to 10 ~ winking both eyes totally for 10 times.
  ~ by counting 1/2 to 10/2 ~ winking both eyes totally for 20 times.
  ~ by counting 1/2/3 to 10/2/3 ~ winking both eyes totally for 30 times
  ~ by counting 1/2/3/4 to 10/2/3/4 ~ winking both eyes totally for 40times.

4. To relieve presbyopia:
~ Holding a name card at 30cm ahead of your eyes.
~ Hanging a calendar on the wall at 300cm ahead of your
   eyes.
~ Read one of the words on the name card first and then
   read a word on the calendar.
~ Every time you need to focus your eyes on the word
   you read and make sure you can read it clearly.
~ If you find it difficult to read the small word on the
   name card clearly, try to take a deep breath and focus
   again.
~ Read the small word on the name card and the big word
   on the calendar alternately in a slow tempo first and
   then speed up.

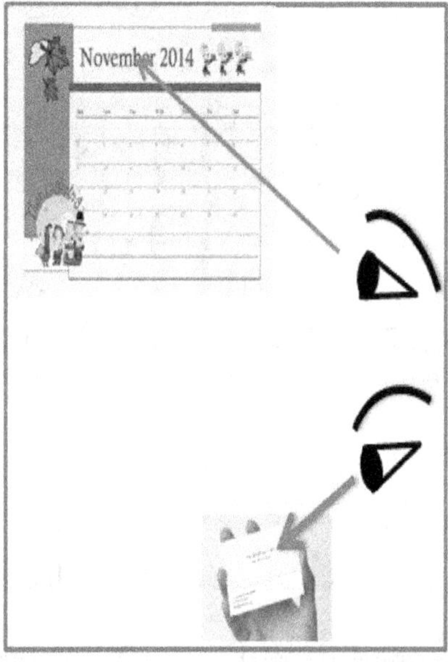

Our eyes, somewhat like a camera, can retain what we
see. Unlike camera, we can only memorize 30% of what
we see. However, our sight is still very significant to our
memory. Constantly training your eyes and maintaining
a good sight can absolutely delay senility.

3) Walk slowly

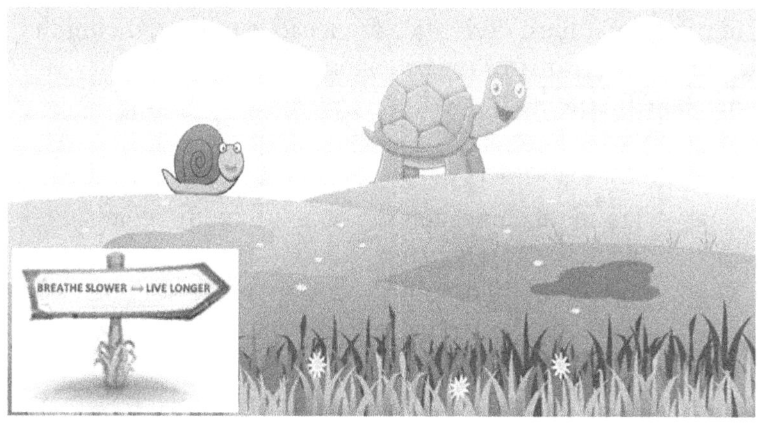

I will take a slow walk in the nearby park for 30 minutes every morning after breakfast.

Walking slowly is good for health, and it can help us to slow down our life.

At this day and age, lots of people are living a life in the fast lane, even though we realized that being busy is no good to our health.

The slower a beings' breathing is, the longer that beings will live.

Comparison of Respiratory Rate in Certain Beings		
Beings	Number of breathing/minute	Life expectancy (years)
Turtle	1~4	200 ~ 1000
Snake	2~3	500 ~ 700
Dog	28~30	15 ~ 16
Rabbit	30~60	5 ~ 10
Human	15 ~ 20	70 ~ 80

You can do it early in the morning like me. Or you can enjoy it after work in which you can soak the early twilight before sunset. Sometimes, do it after dinner to try experiencing the evening breeze of fresh, garden air fanned across your cheeks. Ah...life is so good!

Hints for walking slowly:

➤ Try to take one step in not less than 8 seconds, and then take another step.

➤ Loosen up your mind and body while walking.

➤ Focus on the feeling of your whole body and your breathing.

➤ You can feel your whole world will then be slowing down.

Results:

● Your breathing will be slowing down gradually.

● Your body will become balanced.

● Your anxiety will be relieved.

Slow art is now becoming a modern trend. "Slow" has become a precious pleasure, and a noble quality life. What hidden behind most people's hearts are their longing for leisure, freedom, calm and harmonious. Slow walking for 30 minutes per day will surely alter your life.

4) Drink enough water

Since drinking enough water is so important to our health, I set a time schedule to remind me to drink water at the proper time every day.

Time	Water	When
07:00	300cc	Get up in the morning
08:00	200cc	After doing exercises
09:30		After slow walking
11:30		Before lunch
14:00		Before tea time
17:00		Before sunset
18:30		Before dinner
20:30		After dinner before sleeping

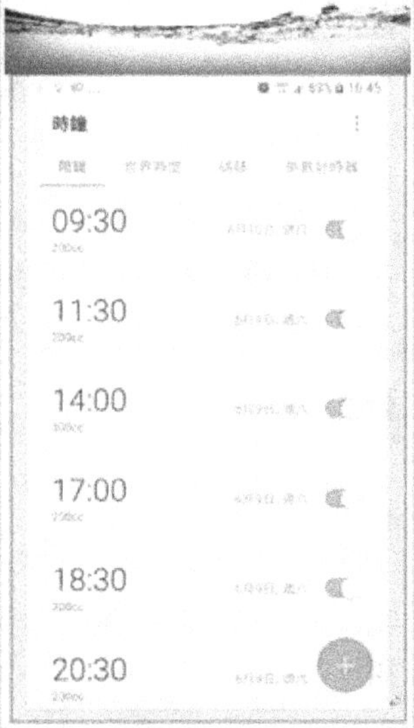

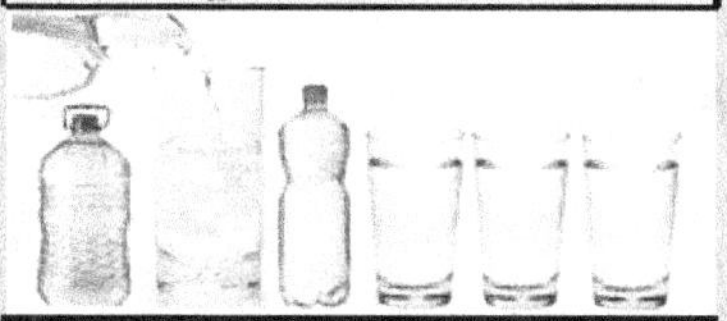

I set alarm clock to my mobile to remind me drinking water.

- Besides eating more fruits and vegetable every day, drinking enough water is essential to avoid constipation.
- How much water is enough? ~
  [Weight (kg) x 30 = minimum cc per day]
  - Age 16 ~ 30 → Weight(kg) x 35 ~ 40
  - Age 31 ~ 54 → Weight(kg) x 30 ~ 35
  - Age 55 ~ 65 → Weight(kg) x 30
  - Age over 65 → Weight(kg) x 25
  - My example: Weight 50kg x 35 = 1750cc

5) Do exercises

I love all sorts of sports and exercises. Every morning, I will spend at least 30 to 40 minutes doing some fitness trainings to start a day.

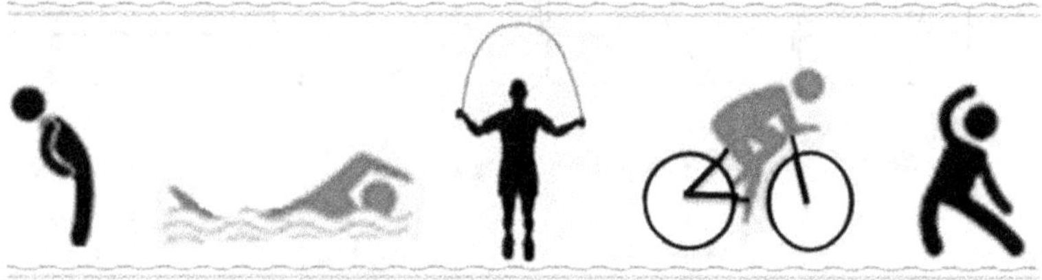

Doing exercises is good for health. And there are many different kinds of exercises and sports you can choose as your daily fitness goals.
Such as:

> Aerobic exercises: Swimming, Cycling, Jumping rope and Jogging
> Sports: Basketball, Tennis, Baseball and Badminton
> Strength trainings: Push-up, Plank, Squat and ABS (abdomen back stretch)
> Kung Fu and Qigong (a system of deep breathing exercises)

I started learning qigong three years ago and find it a very special exercise which can rehabilitate our physical strength as well as delay senility.

I would list out and explain in detail the similarities and differences between sports and qigong as below. It can assist you to understand why qigong is seemlier for us to practice especially when we are comparatively in a poor health status.

Characteristics of qigong:

Comparison of qigong and others exercises		
results	qigong	exercises and sports
become heathier	✓	✓
stengthen muscles	✓	✓
sweating	✓	✓
increasing heart rate	✓	✓
breathe heavily	X	✓
tired	X	✓
sore muscle	X	✓

> ➢ Sweating →
> Qigong is an amazing exercise that I only need to do it very slowly, easily, and seemingly effortlessly, but it can make me sweat all over in a short time. While I am practicing the moves of qigong in a rhythmic-breathing way, I can feel sweat slowly dripping down from my head to my neck, and unceasingly trickling down my back and my whole body. When I am doing other low rhythm exercises, I will not be sweating like this.

> ➢ Increasing heart rate →
> I can hardly feel that my heart rate is increasing during practicing qigong. But when I have finished the qigong moves, my heart beat was measured at about 130 per minutes. Indeed, qigong exercise can also achieve the standard exercise heart rate as other intensive trainings do.

> ➢ Breathing heavily →
> When doing some aerobic exercises or sports, it often needs to breathe heavily, contrary to these intensive trainings; qigong allows me to breathe easily throughout the practice.

> Tired & sore muscle →
> Doing exercise such as strength training or aerobics, sometimes I will be very tired and get sore muscle the next day. However, qigong will not make me feel tired even if I continuously practicing for one hour. It is because our rhythmic breathing can allow the oxygen going through our internal organs as well as the whole body during practicing.

Relationship between our organs, our senses and the whole body

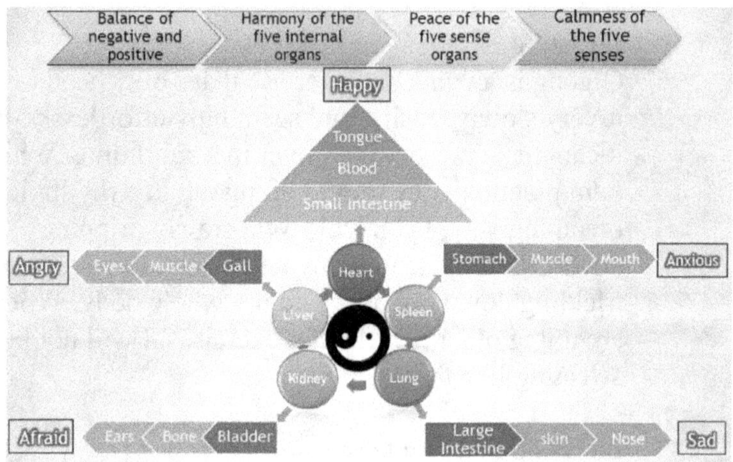

> Our important internal organs: Heart, Spleen, Lung, Kidney and Liver. These five organs are intimately related to each other.

> Heart: Our heart is closely related to our small intestine, blood, and tongue. If you have a strong heart, you will be happy all the time.

> Spleen: Our spleen is closely related to our stomach, muscle, and mouth. If your spleen getting problems, you will easily be anxious.

> Lung: Our lung is closely related with our large intestine, skin, and nose. If your lung is not healthy, you will always feel sad.

> Kidney: Our kidney is closely related with our bladder, bone, and ears. If you have a healthy kidney, you will not easily panic.

> Liver: Our liver is closely related with our gall, muscle, and eyes. If your liver is good enough, you will not easily get angry.

If you can attentively be taking care of your five internal organs, they will be working together cooperatively for you, thus to thoroughly offer you the overall balance, harmony, peace and calmness in all areas of your health.

6) Keep early hours

Studies show that those who identified as early sleepers, who fall asleep before 23:00, reported feeling healthier and worrying less than their night owl counterparts.

I made being an early sleeper a habit when I was in my mid-30s. Persevering to sleep early because I found sleeping can heal my body. Whenever I was feeling unwell like having headache, stomachache, toothache, abdominal pain or period pains etc., just went sleeping for a couple of hours, all those symptoms would be soothed.

Researchers found that sleeping can also help to improve your mood and memory. Moreover, it can calm your flu, for a special brain protein will enhance your body healing power during sleeping, and thus speed its recovery.

Since our body have twelve meridians, the ancient Chinese divided one day into twelve 2-hour periods. Let's look at the below clock and you can find the twelve meridians are relatively corresponding to the twelve 12-hour periods of the day. By knowing when these meridians operate in which periods, we can recognize a more efficient way to keep good health.

Two of the most important 2-hour periods related to sleeping will be explained as below:

1. Gallbladder meridian: (Operating period : 23:00 ~ 1:00)
    This is the significant period of human metabolic, so you must take a good rest.

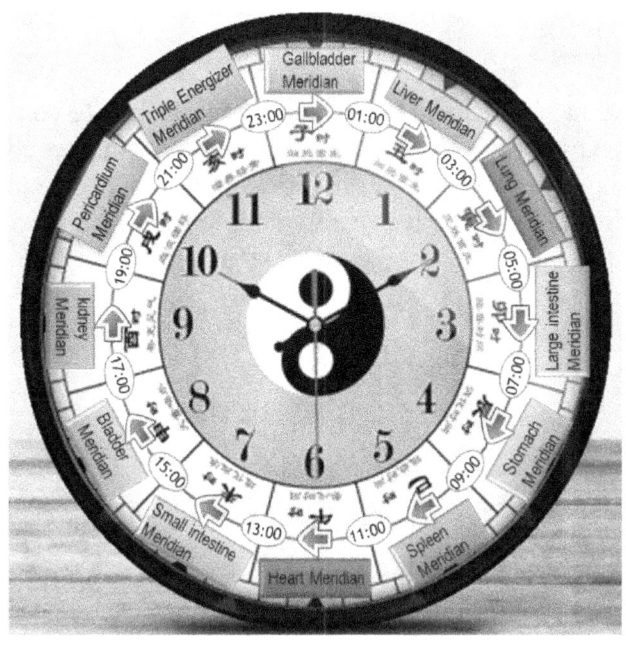

2. Liver meridian: (Operating period : 1:00 ~ 3:00)
   Liver operation period ~ you must take a good rest.
   Liver takes responsibility of filtration of blood toxins
   in the detoxification process at this period. If you
   always stay up late and unable to fall asleep before
   1:00, you are susceptible to hepatitis.

Being an early sleeper is advantageous, so don't
hesitate to make it your habit. Success to do so may
result in positively affecting your kids to follow your
habit in their early life.

7) Set a goal

We all have dreams. Do you want your dreams to come true? One of my spiritual mentors shared with me about setting a goal every night before falling asleep. She has guided me to doing it in a very simple way. And I would like to share with you the major steps of it in the following picture.

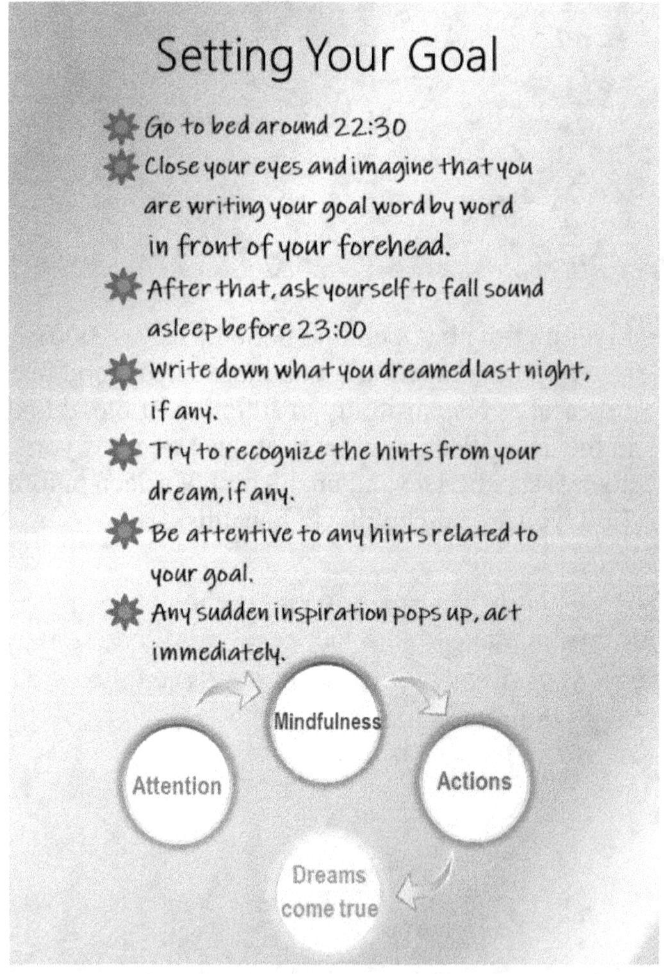

- ➢ Write down on your notebook any goal arising in your mind.
- ➢ Set one goal will be enough for every night.
- ➢ Record all the goals you have set including dates.
- ➢ Most importantly, move on right away upon receiving many hints and inspirations.

In my experience, "setting a goal before sleeping" is indeed, a habit that worth to create. It can lead you to a brand new magnetic field, which is so-called a parallel universe.

8) Complete the worksheet and make notes

- ➢ To supporting you to carry out and stick to this 8-thing plan, I designed the following worksheet for you.

- ➢ You can record and check your results of the previous day by filling in this worksheet. You can also jot down something about the difficulties or failure of carrying out these habits.

Here is a sample of my record and notes for your reference.

Date: Jun 14

Mon ☐ Tue ☐ Wed ☐
Thu ☐ Fri ☑ Sat ☐
Sun ☐

Worksheet

Eight Things Lead You to a Healthier and Easier Life

	✓/X	00:06 ~23:00
Stretch in bed	✓	06:40
Exercise your eyes	✓	06:50
Do exercises	✓	07:00
Walk slowly	X	X
Drink enough water	X	07:00 ~20:30
Keep early hours	X	23:00
Set a goal	✓	23:00
Complete the worksheet and make notes	✓	08:30 Jun 15

Notes :~

1. missed slow walking ~ heavy rain
2. drank too much soup and juice at the party, not enough water for
3. the day
4.
5.

I joined my best friend Irene's birthday party and got home late last night. I shared with her my 30-day plan about making the 8 things as my habit. Although I failed to complete the 8 things in my worksheet, spending a precious time with Irene is wonderful. And I'm sure that I can successfully accomplish my 8-thing plan from today. Keep it up!

Day __1__ of 30 days

Day 1

Target	Done ✓/✗	Time 00:06 ~23:00
Stretch in bed		
Exercise your eyes		
Do exercises		
Walk slowly		
Drink enough water		
Keep early hours		
Set a goal		
Complete the worksheet and make notes		

Notes:~

1.
2.
3.
4.
5.

Day ___ of 30 days

Day 2

<table>
<tr><td colspan="3">Date: _______________</td><td colspan="2">Mon ☐ Tue ☐ Wed ☐
Thu ☐ Fri ☐ Sat ☐
Sun ☐</td></tr>
</table>

Worksheet

Eight Things Lead You to a Healthier and Easier Life

Target	Done ✓/✗	Time 00:06 ~23:00
Stretch in bed		
Exercise your eyes		
Do exercises		
Walk slowly		
Drink enough water		
Keep early hours		
Set a goal		
Complete the worksheet and make notes		

Notes:~

1.
2.
3.
4.
5.

Day 3

Date: ___________

Worksheet

Eight Things Lead You to a Healthier and Easier Life

Target	Done ✓/X	Time 00:06 ~23:00
Stretch in bed		
Exercise your eyes		
Do exercises		
Walk slowly		
Drink enough water		
Keep early hours		
Set a goal		
Complete the worksheet and make notes		

Notes:~

1.

2.

3.

4.

5.

Day 4

Worksheet

Date: _____________

Mon ☐ Tue ☐ Wed ☐
Thu ☐ Fri ☐ Sat ☐
Sun ☐

Eight Things Lead You to a Healthier and Easier Life

Target	Done ✓/✗	Time 00:06 ~23:00
Stretch in bed		
Exercise your eyes		
Do exercises		
Walk slowly		
Drink enough water		
Keep early hours		
Set a goal		
Complete the worksheet and make notes		

Notes:~

1.
2.
3.
4.
5.

Day 5

<table>
<tr><td>Date: ___________</td><td>**Worksheet**</td><td>Mon ☐ Tue ☐ Wed ☐
Thu ☐ Fri ☐ Sat ☐
Sun ☐</td></tr>
</table>

Eight Things Lead You to a Healthier and Easier Life

Target	Done ✓/✗	Time 00:06 ~23:00
Stretch in bed		
Exercise your eyes		
Do exercises		
Walk slowly		
Drink enough water		
Keep early hours		
Set a goal		
Complete the worksheet and make notes		

Notes : ~

1.
2.
3.
4.
5.

Day 6

Worksheet

Mon ☐ Tue ☐ Wed ☐
Thu ☐ Fri ☐ Sat ☐
Sun ☐

Eight Things Lead You to a Healthier and Easier Life

Target	Done ✓/✗	Time 00:06 ~23:00
Stretch in bed		
Exercise your eyes		
Do exercises		
Walk slowly		
Drink enough water		
Keep early hours		
Set a goal		
Complete the worksheet and make notes		

Notes:~

1.
2.
3.
4.
5.

Day 7

<table>
<tr><td>Date: ___________</td><td>**Worksheet**</td><td>Mon ☐ Tue ☐ Wed ☐
Thu ☐ Fri ☐ Sat ☐
Sun ☐</td></tr>
</table>

Eight Things Lead You to a Healthier and Easier Life

Target	Done ✓/✗	Time 00:06 ~23:00
Stretch in bed		
Exercise your eyes		
Do exercises		
Walk slowly		
Drink enough water		
Keep early hours		
Set a goal		
Complete the worksheet and make notes		

Notes:~

1.
2.
3.
4.
5.

Day 8

<table>
<tr><td>Date:_______________</td><td># Worksheet</td><td>Mon ☐ Tue ☐ Wed ☐
Thu ☐ Fri ☐ Sat ☐
Sun ☐</td></tr>
</table>

Worksheet

Eight Things Lead You to a Healthier and Easier Life

Target	Done ✓/✗	Time 00:06 ~23:00
Stretch in bed		
Exercise your eyes		
Do exercises		
Walk slowly		
Drink enough water		
Keep early hours		
Set a goal		
Complete the worksheet and make notes		

Notes:~

1.
2.
3.
4.
5.

Day 9

Target	Done ✓/✗	Time 00:06 ~23:00
Stretch in bed		
Exercise your eyes		
Do exercises		
Walk slowly		
Drink enough water		
Keep early hours		
Set a goal		
Complete the worksheet and make notes		

Notes:~

1.

2.

3.

4.

5.

Day 10

<table>
<tr><td>Date:________</td><td>Worksheet</td><td>Mon ☐ Tue ☐ Wed ☐
Thu ☐ Fri ☐ Sat ☐
Sun ☐</td></tr>
</table>

Worksheet
Eight Things Lead You to a Healthier and Easier Life

Target	Done ✓/✗	Time 00:06 ~23:00
Stretch in bed		
Exercise your eyes		
Do exercises		
Walk slowly		
Drink enough water		
Keep early hours		
Set a goal		
Complete the worksheet and make notes		

Notes:~
1.
2.
3.
4.
5.

Day 11

<table>
<tr><td>Date: _______________</td><td colspan="2" align="center"># Worksheet</td><td>Mon ☐ Tue ☐ Wed ☐
Thu ☐ Fri ☐ Sat ☐
Sun ☐</td></tr>
</table>

Eight Things Lead You to a Healthier and Easier Life

Target	Done ✓/X	Time 00:06 ~23:00
Stretch in bed		
Exercise your eyes		
Do exercises		
Walk slowly		
Drink enough water		
Keep early hours		
Set a goal		
Complete the worksheet and make notes		

Notes : ~

1.
2.
3.
4.
5.

Day 12

<table>
<tr><td>Date: _______________</td><td># Worksheet</td><td>Mon ☐ Tue ☐ Wed ☐
Thu ☐ Fri ☐ Sat ☐
Sun ☐</td></tr>
</table>

Worksheet

Eight Things Lead You to a Healthier and Easier Life

Target	Done ✓/X	Time 00:06 ~ 23:00
Stretch in bed		
Exercise your eyes		
Do exercises		
Walk slowly		
Drink enough water		
Keep early hours		
Set a goal		
Complete the worksheet and make notes		

Notes:~

1.
2.
3.
4.
5.

Day 13

<table>
<tr><td>Date: _____________</td><td colspan="2" align="center">Worksheet</td><td>Mon ☐ Tue ☐ Wed ☐
Thu ☐ Fri ☐ Sat ☐
Sun ☐</td></tr>
</table>

Eight Things Lead You to a Healthier and Easier Life

Target	Done ✓/✗	Time 00:06 ~23:00
Stretch in bed		
Exercise your eyes		
Do exercises		
Walk slowly		
Drink enough water		
Keep early hours		
Set a goal		
Complete the worksheet and make notes		

Notes:~

1.
2.
3.
4.
5.

Day 14

<table>
<tr><td colspan="3">Mon ☐ Tue ☐ Wed ☐</td></tr>
</table>

Date: ___________

Worksheet

Eight Things Lead You to a Healthier and Easier Life

Target	Done ✓ / X	Time 00:06 ~23:00
Stretch in bed		
Exercise your eyes		
Do exercises		
Walk slowly		
Drink enough water		
Keep early hours		
Set a goal		
Complete the worksheet and make notes		

Mon ☐ Tue ☐ Wed ☐ Thu ☐ Fri ☐ Sat ☐ Sun ☐

Notes:~

1.

2.

3.

4.

5.

Day 15

Worksheet

Date: ________________

Mon ☐ Tue ☐ Wed ☐
Thu ☐ Fri ☐ Sat ☐
Sun ☐

Eight Things Lead You to a Healthier and Easier Life

Target	Done ✓/✗	Time 00:06 ~23:00
Stretch in bed		
Exercise your eyes		
Do exercises		
Walk slowly		
Drink enough water		
Keep early hours		
Set a goal		
Complete the worksheet and make notes		

Notes:~

1.
2.
3.
4.
5.

Day __15__ of 30 days

Day 16

<table>
<tr><td>Date:</td><td colspan="2"></td><td>Mon ☐ Tue ☐ Wed ☐
Thu ☐ Fri ☐ Sat ☐
Sun ☐</td></tr>
</table>

Worksheet

Eight Things Lead You to a Healthier and Easier Life

Target	Done ✓/X	Time 00:06 ~23:00
Stretch in bed		
Exercise your eyes		
Do exercises		
Walk slowly		
Drink enough water		
Keep early hours		
Set a goal		
Complete the worksheet and make notes		

Notes:~

1.
2.
3.
4.
5.

Day 17

Worksheet

Date:_______________

Mon ☐ Tue ☐ Wed ☐
Thu ☐ Fri ☐ Sat ☐
Sun ☐

Eight Things Lead You to a Healthier and Easier Life

Target	Done ✓/X	Time 00:06 ~23:00
Stretch in bed		
Exercise your eyes		
Do exercises		
Walk slowly		
Drink enough water		
Keep early hours		
Set a goal		
Complete the worksheet and make notes		

Notes:~

1.

2.

3.

4.

5.

Day 18

<table>
<tr><td>Date: __________</td><td colspan="2">## Worksheet</td><td>Mon ☐ Tue ☐ Wed ☐
Thu ☐ Fri ☐ Sat ☐
Sun ☐</td></tr>
</table>

Worksheet

Eight Things Lead You to a Healthier and Easier Life

Target	Done ✓/X	Time 00:06 ~23:00
Stretch in bed		
Exercise your eyes		
Do exercises		
Walk slowly		
Drink enough water		
Keep early hours		
Set a goal		
Complete the worksheet and make notes		

Notes:~

1.
2.
3.
4.
5.

Day 18 of 30 days

Day 19

Date: _______________

Worksheet

Mon ☐ Tue ☐ Wed ☐
Thu ☐ Fri ☐ Sat ☐
Sun ☐

Eight Things Lead You to a Healthier and Easier Life

Target	Done ✓/✗	Time 00:06 ~23:00
Stretch in bed		
Exercise your eyes		
Do exercises		
Walk slowly		
Drink enough water		
Keep early hours		
Set a goal		
Complete the worksheet and make notes		

Notes:~

1.
2.
3.
4.
5.

Day 21

Date:_____________

Worksheet

Mon ☐ Tue ☐ Wed ☐
Thu ☐ Fri ☐ Sat ☐
Sun ☐

Eight Things Lead You to a Healthier and Easier Life

Target	Done ✓/✗	Time 00:06~23:00
Stretch in bed		
Exercise your eyes		
Do exercises		
Walk slowly		
Drink enough water		
Keep early hours		
Set a goal		
Complete the worksheet and make notes		

Notes:~

1.

2.

3.

4.

5.

Day 21 of 30 days

Day 22

<table>
<tr><td>Date: ___________</td><td>**Worksheet**</td><td>Mon ☐ Tue ☐ Wed ☐
Thu ☐ Fri ☐ Sat ☐
Sun ☐</td></tr>
</table>

Eight Things Lead You to a Healthier and Easier Life

Target	Done ✓/✗	Time 00:06 ~23:00
Stretch in bed		
Exercise your eyes		
Do exercises		
Walk slowly		
Drink enough water		
Keep early hours		
Set a goal		
Complete the worksheet and make notes		

Notes:~

1.
2.
3.
4.
5.

Day 23

Date:_____________

Worksheet

Mon ☐ Tue ☐ Wed ☐
Thu ☐ Fri ☐ Sat ☐
Sun ☐

Eight Things Lead You to a Healthier and Easier Life

Target	Done ✓/✗	Time 00:06 ~23:00
Stretch in bed		
Exercise your eyes		
Do exercises		
Walk slowly		
Drink enough water		
Keep early hours		
Set a goal		
Complete the worksheet and make notes		

Notes:~

1.

2.

3.

4.

5.

Day 24

<table>
<tr><td>Date: ___________</td><td>**Worksheet**</td><td>Mon ☐ Tue ☐ Wed ☐
Thu ☐ Fri ☐ Sat ☐
Sun ☐</td></tr>
</table>

Worksheet

Eight Things Lead You to a Healthier and Easier Life

Target	Done ✓/✗	Time 00:06 ~23:00
Stretch in bed		
Exercise your eyes		
Do exercises		
Walk slowly		
Drink enough water		
Keep early hours		
Set a goal		
Complete the worksheet and make notes		

Notes:~

1.
2.
3.
4.
5.

Day 25

Worksheet

Eight Things Lead You to a Healthier and Easier Life

Mon ☐ Tue ☐ Wed ☐
Thu ☐ Fri ☐ Sat ☐
Sun ☐

Target	Done ✓/X	Time 00:06 ~23:00
Stretch in bed		
Exercise your eyes		
Do exercises		
Walk slowly		
Drink enough water		
Keep early hours		
Set a goal		
Complete the worksheet and make notes		

Notes:~

1.

2.

3.

4.

5.

Day 26

<table>
<tr><td>Date: ___________</td><td>Worksheet</td><td>Mon ☐ Tue ☐ Wed ☐
Thu ☐ Fri ☐ Sat ☐
Sun ☐</td></tr>
</table>

Eight Things Lead You to a Healthier and Easier Life

Target	Done ✓/✗	Time 00:06 ~23:00
Stretch in bed		
Exercise your eyes		
Do exercises		
Walk slowly		
Drink enough water		
Keep early hours		
Set a goal		
Complete the worksheet and make notes		

Notes:~

1.
2.
3.
4.
5.

Day 27

<table>
<tr><td>Date: ___________</td><td colspan="2">Worksheet</td><td>Mon ☐ Tue ☐ Wed ☐
Thu ☐ Fri ☐ Sat ☐
Sun ☐</td></tr>
</table>

Worksheet

Eight Things Lead You to a Healthier and Easier Life

Target	Done ✓/✗	Time 00:06~23:00
Stretch in bed		
Exercise your eyes		
Do exercises		
Walk slowly		
Drink enough water		
Keep early hours		
Set a goal		
Complete the worksheet and make notes		

Notes:~

1.
2.
3.
4.
5.

Date: _______________

Worksheet

Mon ☐ Tue ☐ Wed ☐
Thu ☐ Fri ☐ Sat ☐
Sun ☐

Eight Things Lead You to a Healthier and Easier Life

Target	Done ✓/X	Time 00:06 ~23:00
Stretch in bed		
Exercise your eyes		
Do exercises		
Walk slowly		
Drink enough water		
Keep early hours		
Set a goal		
Complete the worksheet and make notes		

Notes:~

1.

2.

3.

4.

5.

Day 29

Date:_______________

Worksheet

Mon ☐ Tue ☐ Wed ☐
Thu ☐ Fri ☐ Sat ☐
Sun ☐

Eight Things Lead You to a Healthier and Easier Life

Target	Done ✓/✗	Time 00:06 ~23:00
Stretch in bed		
Exercise your eyes		
Do exercises		
Walk slowly		
Drink enough water		
Keep early hours		
Set a goal		
Complete the worksheet and make notes		

Notes:~

1.

2.

3.

4.

5.

Day 30

Date: _______________

Worksheet

Mon ☐ Tue ☐ Wed ☐
Thu ☐ Fri ☐ Sat ☐
Sun ☐

Eight Things Lead You to a Healthier and Easier Life

Target	Done ✓/✗	Time 00:06 ~23:00
Stretch in bed		
Exercise your eyes		
Do exercises		
Walk slowly		
Drink enough water		
Keep early hours		
Set a goal		
Complete the worksheet and make notes		

Notes:~

1.

2.

3.

4.

5.

➢ To borrow from Dr. Maxwell Maltz:

(1)

> "It takes 21 days to develop a habit."
> ~ Dr. Maxwell Maltz ~

➢ Some people believe that it would take much longer time to developing a habit. Other than the 21-day habit formation theory by Dr. Maxwell Maltz, some studies say that it takes an average of 66 days, or even longer, to create a new habit.

(2)

> "Accept yourself as you are. Otherwise you will never see opportunity. You will not feel free to move toward it; you will feel you are not deserving"
> ~ Dr. Maxwell Maltz ~

➢ But don't panic. According to Dr. Maxwell Maltz's guiding, you'd better accept yourself as you are.
➢ Despite others can get something done in 21 days, you can choose to achieve your own distinct result in a particular period. The reason is that you are unique and special in your own way.
➢ No matter it takes 21 days or 66 days or even longer, you should give yourself more time to enjoy and appreciate this surprising "creation" chance.

Endnotes

I was fortunate enough to get the chance recognizing many amazing habits, which were originated from the Human New World founded by my spiritual mentor Doris C. Y. Chung. Upon further discussions with her, I would be glad to share more about her theories of "creation" in my next book.

www.ingramcontent.com/pod-product-compliance
Lightning Source LLC
Chambersburg PA
CBHW070049260726
48658CB00002B/800